Fasting Diet

Fasting Diet Recipes for Healthy Weight Loss

Erica Mauldin and Laurie R. Dean

Table of Contents

Introduction

The fasting diet, often referred to as intermittent fasting or the 5:2 plan, continues to increase in popularity as dieters continue to learn more about the benefits of this diet plan. Since it skips all the ridiculous restrictions that come with most other diets and allows you to eat want you want five days a week, many find that lack of restrictions sufficient compensation for the two fasting days that allow only 500 calories per day for women and 600 per day for men. Of course, those fasting days mean that you are severely limited in the amount of calories you can consume, so you have to find good recipes that you can use to ensure you have plenty of energy on fasting days. It is also important to find great dishes that will keep you feeling full, even though they are low in calories.

If you want to enjoy the best fasting diet results, it is essential to stick to the calorie guidelines on the two fasting days. However, sometimes it is difficult to find low calories recipes that taste great and fasting diet recipes that are easy on the stomach on the fasting days. To help you stick to your intermittent diet, we have compiled a book full of great fasting weight loss recipes that taste great while helping you stick to your intermittent fasting weight loss plan. From breakfast recipes to great main dishes, you will find something delicious to try for any meal. You can choose from the wide selection of recipes, building your own meal plans for your fasting days. In fact, with all the wonderful recipes available, you will not have to worry about getting bored on fasting days. These recipes taste so great that you will probably end up making them even on non-fasting days. Even if your family is not on the fasting diet with you, they are sure to enjoy these tasty recipes as well.

You will also find a section full of snacks and desserts. Just because you are on a fasting day does not mean that you have to skip on snacks or a healthy sweet treat. The snacks and desserts are low calorie and super delicious, so you can satisfy your cravings, even on your fasting days. The salad, soup and sandwich section is packed with soups that are easy on the stomach, satisfying and low calorie salads and tasty sandwiches that will help you stick to your calorie guidelines for the day. We have also added in helpful calorie information for each of the recipes. This way you can easily keep track of the calories you eat on your fasting days, allowing you to stick to your calorie restrictions without a problem.

Fasting weight loss is possible, and while you do not have to count calories most of the time, counting calories is important on those two fasting days each week. With this cookbook you'll be able to find great recipes that are low in calories so you eat well while sticking to those calorie restrictions. You'll even find a helpful meal plan at the end of the cookbook that will help you organize your meals as you get started with the fasting diet. If you are new to the fasting weight loss plan, you will also find a section that gives you the essential information on intermittent fasting, as well as information on the top benefits of following an intermittent fasting diet.

Chapter 1: What is Intermittent Fasting?

Intermittent fasting continues to grow in popularity, but if you are just getting started with the fasting diet, it is important to understand this diet, as well as how it works. This way you have a better understanding of how to use these fasting diet recipes in your fasting weight loss diet. Going on a diet without understanding how it works will set you up for failure from the start, so take the time to become more familiar with the diet and the science behind it. Here is a closer look at the intermittent diet, how it works, as well as other important information you should know as you embark on this new diet.

What is It?

Often known as the 5:2 diet, intermittent fasting is an eating plan that has you restrict the amount of calories you consume two days each week while eating normally on all the other days. For five days each week you can eat normally, but on the other two days, you will need to severely restrict your caloric intake. Women should only take in 500 calories on fasting days and men should only have about 600 calories on those days.

Severely restricting your calorie intake a couple times a week helps you to reduce overall calorie intake each week, even when you are eating normally on other days. This helps with weight loss and offers a number of other excellent benefits as well, which we will discuss in the next chapter.

It is important to note that the fasting days should not be done consecutively. For example, if you fast on a Monday, then you should not fast on Tuesday. Break up your fasting days, such as fasting on Wednesdays and Saturdays or fasting on Mondays and Wednesdays.

Intermittent Fasting vs Alternate Day Fasting

You may have heard of another diet known as the Alternate Day Fasting Diet. It is similar, but not quite the same as intermittent fasting. Instead of only fasting for two days a week, which you do on the intermittent fasting weight loss plan, the Alternate Day Fasting plan requires you to fast every other day. Of course, even if you are using the Alternate Day Fasting plan, you could still use these great fasting diet recipes to help you out on fasting days.

The Science Behind The Intermittent Fasting Diet

Some evidence and scientific research does show that the intermittent fasting diet does provide results. According to studies, constantly eating the same amount every day puts a strain on your body and it keeps levels of Insulin-like Growth Factor 1 (IGF-1) higher than they should be as adults. Unfortunately, high levels of this growth hormone may increase the risk of certain medical problems. Fasting a couple days a week is supposed to reduce the levels of this hormone, allowing the body to repair itself better while reducing your risk of certain diseases.

Today, human studies have been done on fasting and according to the studies, as long as you have two fasting days each week, you can eat normal foods on the other days and still enjoy weight loss and improved health. While you still want to avoid eating high fat, processed foods regularly, the studies show that you can indulge from time to time as long as you give your body those two fasting days each week to work on repairing itself.

What Makes the Diet Popular?

One of the main reasons for the popularity of the intermittent fasting diet is how easy it is to stick to it.

Yes, you are cutting the calories you eat each week, but it is easier to stick to this diet because on the other days, you get to enjoy eating a normal diet. Even though fasting days make leave you feeling a bit hungry, you still know that you can enjoy your favorite foods on the other days, so it is easy to stick to this diet, unlike many other diets.

While you might think that you would want to binge after a fasting day, studies done on the fasting diet shows that most people do not end up binging after a day of fasting. The studies show that generally people will eat approximately 110% of the calories their body needs, which is okay because of the fasting days. Fasting helps teach your body when you are really hungry, so retraining the body keeps you from indulging when you are not really hungry. This keeps you from binge eating after fasting days.

Some people thinking that eating too little on a single day may make the body start storing up fat because it thinks it is starving. While a regularly diet that drastically reduced calories may cause this problem, as well as other unhealthy side effects, restricting calories only on fasting days will not cause this problem. On the other five days, you are still eating plenty of calories so your body will not be tricked into thinking it is starving. The diet works for most people, but of course, it is always important to talk to your physician before starting this or any other type of diet or exercise plan. This is especially important for those who have medical conditions.

Chapter 2: Benefits of Intermittent Fasting

The fasting diet, which includes intermittent fasting, offers a number of excellent benefits. Many studies support the benefits of this diet, which is why it continues to be a popular option for individuals that want to lose weight or enjoy a healthier lifestyle. The following are just a few of the benefits you can enjoy when following an intermittent fasting diet.

Benefit #1 – Longer Life

One benefit of the fasting diet is the ability to enjoy a longer life. Studies have shown that regularly fasting helps to reduce many different health risks, which increases your longevity. Reducing caloric intake significantly has been proven to extend the lifespan of animals and studies show that this works for humans as well.

Benefit #2 – Easy to Follow

Another top benefit of following this diet is how easy it is to follow. Many good diets fail because they are difficult to follow. While a diet may have science to back it up, if people are not able to stick to it, it will not provide results. With the fasting diet, the ability to eat normally most of the time makes it a diet that most people find easy to follow. A diet that is easy to follow offers the best results, since it can be turned into a lifestyle instead of a short-term diet.

Benefit #3 – Improved Fitness

Although some people say that fasting will make you burn muscles when you work out, when on this intermittent fasting plan, this is not the case. In fact, when training while following this diet, you can end up with a better anabolic response to feeding after workouts, improve protein synthesis and improve metabolic adaptations, which result in improved performance when working out. On fast days, your workouts will help you burn more fat, ensuring that you burn off fat while you are working to lose weight.

Benefit #4 – Improved Mood

Some studies show that adults may enjoy better moods when they follow a fasting diet. Many people who have been studied while participating in intermittent fasting plans have reported that they are able to concentrate better, sleep better and they enjoy greater energy levels as well. This helps improve their overall sense of wellbeing.

Benefit #5 – Reduced Risk of Serious Health Conditions

Following the 5:2 fasting diet helps you maintain a healthy weight, which is important, since obesity causes so many health conditions today. Not only will it help reduce your risk of health conditions related to obesity, but it will also help you to reduce your risk for many other diseases as well, such as heart disease, cancer and diabetes.

Benefit #4 – Enjoy What You Love

So many diet plans fail because it is no fun to have all your favorite foods restricted. Life is too short to always eat food you do not like. With the fasting diet, you still get to enjoy the foods that you love. It does not make you feel like you have too many restrictions. Many delicious foods are available and can be enjoyed in moderation. This diet allows you to enjoy eating tasty food favorites as long as you stick to the days of fasting each week.

With all these excellent benefits, it is easy to see why intermittent fasting has become one of the most popular forms of dieting today. It is easy to follow, allows you to enjoy favorite foods and helps you to prevent health problems in the future as well. You can even work towards a longer life when you follow this diet. Many studies have been done on the fasting diet, so science is there to back up the findings if you are considering the diet.

Chapter 3: Fasting Diet Breakfast Recipes

On your fasting day, you want to start out the day with a healthy, filling, low calorie breakfast. Since you can only eat 500-600 calories per day (depending on if you are a man or woman), you need to make your calories count. If you eat empty calories for breakfast, you will have a tough time fighting off hunger throughout your day. Start the day right with a low calorie breakfast that will fill you up. The key is to eat foods that pack a great nutritional punch while making you feel full. This chapter includes some of the best fasting diet breakfast recipes. They are easy on your stomach and they will fill you up, but best of all, they are low in calories and delightfully scrumptious too.

Berry Blend and Banana Breakfast Smoothie Recipe

With delicious breakfast smoothie, you will be able to keep those energy levels up throughout the day. The smoothie is low in calories and ensures you get excellent nutrition from the blend of fruits included. All the berries in this smoothie even makes sure that you enjoy a nice dose of antioxidants to start your day. It is easy to whip up this smoothie, even on days that you do not have a lot of time. Inspired by a recipe from the 5:2 Fasting Diet Plan, this smoothie only has 126 calories and an unexpected twist when you drink it.

What You'll Need:

- 1 cup of ice cubes

- 2 ripe bananas, sliced

- 1 cup of fresh or frozen blueberries

- ¼ teaspoon of cinnamon powder

- 1 cup of fresh or frozen raspberries

- 3 teaspoon of raw honey

- 1 cup of unsweetened apple juice

- 1/8 teaspoon of nutmeg

How to Make It:

Wash all the berries before using them. Peel and slice the bananas. Place the ice, berries and bananas in the blender. Drizzle the honey on top, add the apple juice and then add the cinnamon and nutmeg. Blend by pulsing until the fruit has been chopped into pieces. Stir up the mixture and then continue blending until you have a smooth, creamy smoothie. Drink and enjoy right away. Makes 2 servings.

Egg and Summer Veggie Omelet Recipe

Some people enjoy eating most of their fasting day calories for breakfast, while others like to save most of them for dinner. This tasty recipe has about 250 calories, which is close to half of your daily calories on a fasting day. Cook it up for a filling, protein packed breakfast. You could even make this delicious omelet for a nice, fast dinner. The eggs give you plenty of protein and you will get important nutrients from the tasty veggies included in the omelet.

What You'll Need:

2 tablespoons of skim milk

3 large eggs

1/3 cup of asparagus spears, chopped

1/3 cup of mushrooms, chopped

1/3 cup of cherry tomatoes, cut in half

1/8 cup of onions, chopped

Pepper and salt to taste

How to Make It:

Start by chopping all the veggies for your omelet. Place the eggs in a medium bowl and add the milk. Beat the eggs, incorporating the milk. Add a bit of pepper and salt and beat into the eggs.

Spray a non-stick skillet with some olive oil cooking spray. Heat to medium heat. Add the onions, asparagus and mushrooms to the skillet and allow to sauté for 4-6 minutes, or until tender. Then, add the cherry tomatoes to the pan, allowing to cook for another minute.

Heat an omelet pan and spray with olive oil cooking spray. Pour eggs into the omelet pan. Cook on medium until the eggs have set enough to flip. Flip and then cook for another couple minutes, ensuring that eggs are fully cook. Place omelet on a plate, fill with the vegetable mixture and fold the omelet over. Enjoy while hot. Makes 1 large omelet.

Egg White and Spinach Omelet Recipe

Since you want to limit the number of calories that you eat for breakfast while ensuring you get enough food to give you energy for your day, this egg white and spinach omelet is a great breakfast recipe for your fasting days. Inspired by a recipe from The Fasting Diet Plan, the entire omelet only has 80 calories, so you can easily stick to your intermittent fasting weight loss plan. The egg whites keep calories low while giving you some protein and the tomatoes and spinach offers plenty of important nutrients. The bit of Parmesan cheese adds flavor to your omelet.

What You'll Need:

1 tablespoon of parmesan cheese, grated

½ cups of finely chopped spinach

3 egg whites

3 medium cherry tomatoes, sliced thinly

Pepper and salt to taste

How to Make It:

In a small bowl, whip the egg whites until well beaten. Add the sliced tomatoes and the chopped spinach to the bowl and mix well. Spray a small skillet with some olive oil cooking spray and heat on medium heat. Add eggs to the skillet and sprinkle with a bit of salt and pepper to taste. Cook until eggs are fully cooked and set. Lower heat and top with the parmesan cheese. Fold the omelet with the cheese inside and place on a plate. Enjoy while it's hot. Makes a single serving.

Tasty Bran Banana Muffins Recipe

For just 97 calories per serving, you can enjoy tasty bran and banana muffins for breakfast. They include apples, bananas and raisins, which give you a nice serving of fruit. The muffins are made with whole wheat flour and wheat bran, which makes the muffins very dense. The great thing about these muffins, which are inspired by a tasty Spark People Recipe is that you can mix them up in just a few minutes and you will have 12 muffins to enjoy throughout the week, even on your fasting days while on the fasting diet.

What You'll Need:

- ½ cup of brown sugar

- 1 medium Granny Smith apple

- 1 cup of crude wheat bran

- ¼ cup of milk (2%)

- ½ teaspoon of vanilla extract

- ½ cup of whole wheat flour

- 1 teaspoon of ground cinnamon

- ¼ cup of raisins

- 1 large egg

- 2 ripe bananas

- 1 teaspoon of baking soda

- ¼ teaspoon of salt

- ½ teaspoon of baking powder

How to Make It:

Preheat your oven to 350F.

Peel the apple and remove the core. Then shred the apple until it is finely shredded. Mash the bananas.

In a large bowl, combine the brown sugar, wheat bran, wheat flour, cinnamon, raisins, baking soda, salt and baking soda. Mix thoroughly. Then, in a medium bowl, combine the milk, vanilla extract, mashed banana and egg, mixing thoroughly. Combine the wet ingredients with the dry ingredients and combine. Avoid over mixing. Then, add the shredded apple to the mix and fold in. Divide the mixture between 12 muffin cups.

Place muffins in the oven and bake on 350F for 20-25 minutes. Muffins should rise and set when they are done. Remove from the oven and allow to cook. Enjoy warm or cool. Recipe makes 12 muffins.

Poached Eggs with Asparagus Breakfast Recipe

This breakfast recipe is super simple and it will not take a lot of time for you to make in the morning. It makes a wonderful light breakfast to eat while on your intermittent diet, but you could eat it for dinner too if you enjoy eggs for dinner. Per serving, you will only be getting about 150 calories, so it fits perfectly into your low calorie fasting days. The white wine vinegar and garlic really adds flavor to this delicious breakfast dish.

What You'll Need

- 4 large eggs
- 32 spears of asparagus
- 4-6 garlic cloves
- 2 tablespoons of white wine vinegar
- Salt and pepper to taste
- 2 tablespoons of olive oil
- 2-3 teaspoons of grated parmesan

How to Make It:

In a large non-stick skillet, heat the olive oil on medium heat. Add the asparagus to the pan and allow to sauté until it begins softening. As the asparagus is cooking, mince the garlic. Once the asparagus is tender, add the minced garlic to the pan, continuing to cook until garlic becomes crisp.

While the asparagus is cooking, bring water to boil in a large pot. Add the white wine vinegar to the water before it comes to a boil. Before adding eggs to water, whisk the water to spread the vinegar throughout. Break 1 egg in a cup and then carefully put the egg in the boiling water. Allow to cook for about 2-3 minutes until egg whites are completely cooked. Remove with a slotted spoon. Repeat with the rest of the eggs.

Serve eggs over the garlic and asparagus, sprinkling with the grated parmesan before serving. Eat while hot. Makes 4 servings.

Blackberry Apple Breakfast Muffins Recipe

When you want a sweet, healthy breakfast, these blackberry apple breakfast muffins make a delightful breakfast. They will quash any cravings for sweets while giving you a nice breakfast that is easy on the stomach. The combination of apple and blackberries is delicious and the recipe is sweetened with just a bit of stevia for added sweetness without adding sugar. Enjoy a muffin for about 180 calories.

What You'll Need:

- 4 tablespoons of baking powder

- 2 apples (any kind)

- 2 eggs

- 8 teaspoons of Stevia

- 2 teaspoons of ground cinnamon

- ½ cup of rapeseed oil

- 1 cup of blackberries

- 1 cup of wholemeal flour, plain

- ½ cup of skim milk

How to Make It:

Preheat the oven to 375 F. Prepare a muffin pan by adding muffin papers to the each muffin hole.

Peel and core the apples, then cut into chunks and place into a food processor. Pulse until roughly chopped. Add the blackberries to the processor and pulse a couple more times until the blackberries are roughly chopped.

In a large bowl, mix the Stevia with the chopped blackberries and apples.

In a medium bowl, sift together the cinnamon, baking powder and flour. In the center, create a well.

In a small bowl, mix the milk, rapeseed oil and the eggs. Whisk together until well combined. Pour the wet ingredients into the well you created in the dry ingredients. Mix until the dry and wet ingredients are combined. Add the fruit to the bowl, mixing without over mixing the batter.

Divide the batter among the 12 muffin cups. Place in the oven and allow to bake at 375 for 20-30 minutes, or until an inserted fork comes out completely clean. Remove muffins from the oven and then place muffins on a wire rack to let them cool. Enjoy warm or cold. Makes 12 servings.

Peanut Butter Chocolate Cold Oatmeal Recipe

Oatmeal always makes an excellent choice for breakfast, since it is packed with stomach filling fiber. Oats are also wonderful for preventing heart disease, so eating oats will fill you up, give you energy and help you reduce your risk of heart disease. This recipe adds cocoa powder and peanut butter to the oats, packing in plenty of great flavor for you to enjoy. The great thing about this cold oatmeal recipe is you can mix it up and place in the refrigerator the night before, not to mention, it only has about 280 calories for each serving. The next morning, you simply grab it from the refrigerator and enjoy.

What You'll Need:

- 2 tablespoons of peanut butter

- 1 cup of oatmeal

- 2 cups of almond milk, unsweetened

- Stevia to taste

- 1 tablespoon of cocoa powder, unsweetened

How to Make It:

In a large bowl, mix the almond milk, cocoa powder and oatmeal together until well combined. Divide the oats among two jars. Place a lid on the jars and place in the refrigerator. Allow to refrigerate at least 8 hours, or overnight. Before eating the oats, stir 1 tablespoon of peanut butter into each jar. Sweeten with Stevia to taste. Enjoy cold. Makes 2 servings.

Chapter 4: Fasting Diet Snacks and Desserts

Even when you are following the fasting diet, sometimes you will need a snack. Even with a small amount of calories allowed on a fasting day, you can still fit in a low calorie snack if you need a little extra boost. You may even get a craving for something sweet on your fasting day and you do not have to skip sweets if they are low in calories. These fasting diet recipes offer great snacks and wonderful desserts that are healthy and tasty. Just make sure you remember to count the calories of your snack or dessert to ensure you do not eat more than the recommended calories on your fasting day. This way you enjoy the most fasting fat loss while still eating some delicious food.

Artichoke and Spinach Dip Recipe

Artichoke and spinach dip is wonderfully delicious and you can even enjoy it when you are on your fasting days, since you can have a serving for less than 75 calories. It only takes a few minutes to prepare it and makes 20 servings, so you can eat it throughout the week or share it with friends and family members. The flavor of this dip, inspired by a Spark People recipe, is incredible and comes from the red pepper flakes, artichokes, garlic, onions and the parmesan cheese that is included. A bit of lemon juice gives the dip a nice zing. It makes a great dip for veggies, which have few calories, so you can enjoy them on your fasting days and have the dip to give them some extra flavor.

What You'll Need:

- ½ teaspoon of oregano

- 2 packages of cream cheese, light (8oz)

- 1/3 cup of parmesan cheese

- 14 oz. bag of frozen artichokes

- ½ teaspoon of red pepper flakes

- Nonstick olive oil cooking spray

- 10 ounces of baby spinach, steamed

- 1 tablespoon of lemon juice

- 2 cloves of garlic, finely minced

- 1 small onion, finely minced

- Pepper and salt to taste

- Chopped tomatoes for garnish

How to Make It:

Spray the inside of a slow cooker with some nonstick olive oil cooking spray.

Heat a small skillet on medium heat, spraying with some cooking spray. Add the onions and garlic to the pan, sautéing them until they are tender, which takes about 4-6 minutes.

In a food processor, place spinach and chop by pulsing a few times. Place artichokes in the processor with the spinach, processing again to chop. Avoid over chopping, since you want a chunky mixture.

Add the spinach and artichoke mixture to the slow cooker. Add the sautéed onions and garlic. Place the red pepper, lemon juice, cream cheese and oregano in the slow cooker as well. Turn slow cooker on low and allow to cook for about 4 hours. After four hours, add the parmesan cheese to the mix and stir. Add a bit of milk if the mixture is too thick. Season to taste with some pepper and salt. Serve warm with veggies of choice, garnishing with some chopped tomatoes if desired. Makes 20 servings.

Glazed and Iced Cinnamon Pineapple Dessert Recipe

Sometimes you just crave dessert and you do not have to give up something sweet when you on a fasting day when you find low calorie desserts like this one. You can have this dessert, inspired by a recipe from BBC Good Food, for just 160 calories. It does not require a lot of effort to make and it is ready in no time as well. It is so delicious that you will want to make this even on days that you are not fasting for your intermittent diet.

What You'll Need:

- 1 pineapple, cut into long wedges (make about 8 wedges)

- Pinch of nutmeg

- 1 lime, juice and zest

- 2 teaspoons of butter

- 2 pinches of cinnamon

- 2 teaspoons of sifted icing sugar

- 2 tablespoons of pure, clear honey

- ¾ cup of fromage frais, low fat

How to Make It:

Start by mixing the nutmeg, cinnamon, 1 tablespoon of the honey, half the lime zest and the lime juice together in a small bowl. Set to the side. Then, in a small bowl, stir together a pinch of cinnamon and the icing sugar into your fromage frais.

In a non-stick skillet, heat the other tablespoon of honey and the butter over high heat. When butter melts, add pineapple, cooking on high and continually turning until the pineapple caramelizes. Add the lime sauce over the pineapple and allow to bubble for several seconds. Toss the pineapple with the lime sauce to glaze the pineapple.

Divide the pineapple among 4 plates. Top pineapple with the rest of the lime zest and add a spoon of the fromage frais mixture to the pineapples as well for dipping. Enjoy while pineapple is warm. Makes 4 servings.

Tasty Veggie and Cheese Stuffed Mushrooms Recipe

Stuffed mushrooms are a delicious snack and this recipe allows you to enjoy the mushrooms without consuming a lot of calories. Portobello mushrooms make great mushrooms for stuffing, so you may want to use them for this recipe. You will get some protein from the cheese and great nutrients from the veggies included in the stuffing. One mushroom (which is a serving) packs nearly 6 grams of protein and has only 79 calories.

What You'll Need:

- 1 clove of garlic, finely diced

- ¼ teaspoon of coriander

- 1 teaspoon of olive oil

- ½ large onion, chopped

- ¼ teaspoon of paprika

- 2 teaspoons of parmesan cheese

- 10 oz. of chopped spinach, frozen

- ½ cup of cheddar cheese

- 6 large mushrooms for stuffing (about 14oz total)

- Pepper and salt to taste

How to Make It:

Start by preheating your oven to 350F.

Carefully clean the mushrooms with a paper towel before using them. Hollow out the caps of the mushrooms to prepare them for stuffing. Spray an 8x8 pan with olive oil cooking spray and then place the mushroom caps in the pan.

In a large non-stick skillet, heat the olive oil over medium heat. When the oil is hot, add the garlic and onions to the oil, allowing the veggies to sauté until they become tender. Add the spinach to the skillet, mixing in with the garlic and onions. Place parmesan and cheddar cheese to the pan, mixing everything up thoroughly. Turn hit on low and continue stirring. Then, add coriander, paprika and pepper and salt to taste to the mixture.

Take the mushroom stuffing off the heat. Carefully divide the mixture among the six mushroom caps.

Place mushrooms in the oven, cooking for 20 minutes at 350 or until your mushrooms reach your desired doneness. Enjoy while warm. Makes six servings.

Almond and Honey Topped Figs Recipe

Figs are such a healthy fruit and this recipe adds almonds and honey to the figs for a healthy, delicious dessert that is ready in just a few minutes. Enjoy this sweet dish for only 150 calories per serving. The Greek yogurt offers some protein and the cinnamon and honey packs in plenty of delicious flavor to your dish.

What You'll Need:

- 2 tablespoons of honey

- 4 tablespoons of Greek yogurt (no fat)

- ½ teaspoon of cinnamon

- 4 ripe figs

- Toasted slivered almonds for garnishing

How to Make It:

To make this tasty dessert, start by cutting all the figs in half. Place four halves on one plate and four halves on a second plate. Spoon half the yogurt over each plate of figs. Drizzle with the honey. Sprinkle each plate of figs with half of the cinnamon. Top with the toasted almonds. Eat immediately and enjoy. Makes 2 servings.

Easy Red Pepper Hummus Recipe

Hummus always makes an excellent snack because it is low in calories and high in dietary fiber. It also offers some protein. The high fiber content makes hummus super satisfying, making it a perfect snack to grab on your fasting days as you are following the fasting weight loss diet. This hummus recipe adds red pepper to the mix, giving you plenty of flavor for only a few calories. A serving is only 33 calories, so pair it up with a handful of veggies.

What You'll Need:

- 4 tablespoons of lemon juice

- 2 cans of garbanzo beans (15.5oz cans), well drained

- 3 tablespoons of tahini

- 6 cloves of garlic, finely minced

- ¼ teaspoon of red pepper flakes

- ½ cup of red bell pepper

How to Make It:

Add the red bell pepper and the garbanzo beans in your food processor. Process until you have a smooth paste. Add the tahini, lemon juice, red pepper flakes and garlic to the food processor. Continue blending until the mixture is completely smooth. Add a little more lemon juice if you need to think the hummus a bit. Enjoy with veggies. Refrigerate for up to 5 days. Makes about 40 servings, so share with the whole family.

Lemon and Blueberry Yogurt Cake Recipe

Who knew that you could enjoy a piece of cake for 115 calories? This delicious cake allows you to have your cake, and eat it too without feeling guilty. It makes the perfect dessert when you want something sweet and tasty while you are on a fasting day. It is delicious and easy on your digestive system. Make the cake for your fasting day and enjoy it all week long!

What You'll Need:

- 8 ounces of Greek yogurt, low fat, plain
- 3 eggs (separated)
- 1 teaspoon of baking powder
- ½ cup of sugar
- 1 cup of blueberries
- ¾ cup of milk (preferably skim)
- 1 tablespoon of applesauce
- 1 cup of self-rising flour
- 1 teaspoon of vanilla
- 1 lemon, zest and juice

How to Make It:

Start by preheating the oven to 350F.

Take an 8inch round or square cake pan and line it with some parchment paper so you will not need to use any cooking spray for the cake.

In a large bowl, mix the sugar, flour and baking powder until well combined. In another medium size bowl, mix the milk, egg yolks, vanilla, yogurt, applesauce, lemon zest and lemon juice. Mix well. Then, add blueberries and fold into the wet ingredients. In a small bowl, place egg whites and whisk until they become fluffy and white.

Make a well in the dry ingredients and then pour the yogurt blueberry mixture into the well, mixing the two together until completely incorporated. Fold egg whites into the mixture, mixing well but avoid over mixing.

Pour cake batter into the prepared pan and place in the oven. Bake at 350F for 30 minutes. Use a toothpick to test the center of the cake. When it comes out almost dry, the cake can be removed from the oven. Remove cake and allow to cool for about 10 minutes. Serve warm. You can also enjoy cold later. Makes 12 servings.

Raspberry Greek Yogurt Chocolate Dessert Recipe

Everyone can use a little chocolate goodness now and then and this raspberry Greek yogurt chocolate dessert is sure to please. You can have a small serving on your fasting day for 160 calories or enjoy a double serving on your non-fasting days, since it makes 12 small servings (or 6 double servings). It tastes wonderful and only takes about 15 minutes of prep time.

What You'll Need:

- 1 cup of dark chocolate

- 2 ¼ cups of Greek yogurt, plain

- ½ cup of fresh raspberries (you can use frozen if you defrost them first)

- 3 tablespoons of honey

- Grated chocolate for garnish

How to Make It:

Take dark chocolate and break into smaller pieces, placing in a bowl that is heatproof. Fill a medium saucepan about halfway with water and bring the water to a boil. Place the bowl on top of the saucepan, ensuring that the bowl doesn't touch the boiling water.

Allow the chocolate to slowly melt in the bowl.

When chocolate is melted, remove from heat and allow to cool for about 9-11 minutes. While the chocolate cools, place raspberries in the bottom of a round 8 inch cake pan. After the chocolate has cooled, mix it with the honey and yogurt. Spoon the mixture over all of the raspberries.

Place the pan in the refrigerator, allowing the dessert to cool for a couple hours. Serve when cool with some grated chocolate on top as a garnish. Enjoy. Makes 12 small servings (or 6 double servings).

Chapter 5: Fasting Diet Main Dishes

For most people, they choose to have dinner as their largest meal on their fasting days. These main dish recipes are perfect for the larger meal of your day. While they make great dinners, you could also eat these dishes for lunch if you prefer to keep your main calorie intake earlier in the day. You will not even feel deprived with these wonderful recipes that are full of flavor and ingredients that fill you up while offering a great nutritional punch. If you are craving Chinese, try the Beef and Veggie Stir Fry recipe or the Teriyaki Grilled Veggie Tofu Kebabs. You will even find a couple pizza recipes on the list, so you can enjoy one of your favorite foods, since these recipes are made over to keep calories low and nutrition high. From Mushroom Garlic Chicken to Spinach and Smoked Salmon Roulade, you are sure to enjoy all of these great fasting diet main dish recipes.

Red Pepper and Chorizo Pilaf Recipe

Finding filling meals that taste great and keep you feeling full and full of energy can be difficult on your fasting days. However, this delicious red pepper and chorizo pilaf only has 237 calories for a serving, which means you can easily stick to your calorie requirements on fasting days. The flavor tastes rich, but the brown rice fills you up and gives you plenty of fiber. Inspired by a recipe from the Intermittent Fasting Guide, you are sure to enjoy all the flavors that come together in this recipe, such as garlic, red peppers, olives, chorizo and smoked paprika.

What You'll Need:

- 5 green olives, pits removed and cut in half

- 1 tablespoon of chopped flat leaf parsley

- ½ tablespoon of tomato puree

- 1 clove of crushed garlic

- 1/8 cup of brown rice, uncooked

- 1 teaspoon of smoked paprika

- 1/8 cup of chorizo, chopped finely

- ¼ cup of red bell pepper, chopped roughly

- ½ cup of chopped canned tomatoes

- ½ cup of chicken stock

How to Make It:

Take a medium saucepan and heat it up on medium high heat. When the pan is hot, add the chopped chorizo to the pan and fry for a couple minutes until the oils start releasing from the sausage. Add the tomato puree, garlic, paprika and onions to the pan, allowing to cook for about four more minutes, or until onion becomes tender. Add red peppers and allow to cook for another two minutes.

Stir chopped tomatoes, chicken stock olives and rice to the pan, sprinkling with a bit of black pepper. Cover the saucepan and allow the mixture to simmer for about 20-25 minutes until the rice absorbs the liquid and becomes tender. Stir from time to time to ensure that rice does not stick to the saucepan. If necessary, you can add a bit more water.

Serve while hot and garnish with chopped parsley. Enjoy! Makes 1 single serving.

Low Cal Turkey Bolognese Recipe

A recipe from London Unattached inspired this tasty recipe that goes wonderfully with your fasting diet when you are on a fasting day. It offers a delicious dish that is low in calories and fat. A single serving of this turkey Bolognese is only 182 calories, so you have plenty of room to eat other foods on your fasting day. Along with delicious turkey, which gives you a nice protein boost, it includes plenty of veggies, such as carrots, celery, tomatoes and onions, as well as some lean bacon.

What You'll Need:

- 4 stalks of celery, chopped finely

- 1 cup of cooked turkey

- 2 medium onions, chopped finely

- 2 teaspoons of Worcester sauce

- 2 teaspoons of olive oil

- 4 cloves of finely chopped garlic

- 2 small carrots, finely chopped

- ½ star anise

- 2 teaspoons of dried oregano

- 3 1/3 cups of canned chopped tomatoes

- ¼ cup of lean bacon, chopped

- 1 cup of vegetable stock

How to Make It:

Add the oil to a saucepan and allow it to warm over medium heat. Add the star anise to the pan and heat in the saucepan for a couple minutes. Add the bacon, carrot, garlic, celery and onion to the pan, allowing to sauté for 6-8 more minutes until veggies become soft. Regularly stir the mixture as it cooks.

When veggies are tender, add the diced turkey and the oregano to the pan. Add the rest of the ingredients to the pan and bring it to a simmer. Allow the mixture to simmer for about 20 minutes. Stir from time to time. If the mixture dries out, add some more water to it. Season with pepper and salt to taste.

Serve the sauce over a single serving of pasta. Top with a small sprinkle of parmesan cheese if desired, but add the calories to the total calories. Eat warm. Makes 6 servings.

Beef and Veggie Stir Fry Recipe

Stir fries are delicious, so you may not think that a stir fry would be suitable for your fasting days. However, with all the veggies, you can create a low calorie, yet filling, stir fry that tastes wonderful and works well even when you are doing your fasting days. It allows you to stick to the low calorie restrictions as you work on getting fasting diet results. The beef ensures you get protein for energy and all the yummy veggies ensure you get important nutrients that your body needs. Each serving of this recipe comes out to about 260 calories.

What You'll Need:

- 2 ½ cups of stir fry beef strips

- ¾ cup of sliced red bell peppers

- ¾ cup of baby sweetcorn, chopped roughly

- ½ cup of chopped sugar snap peas

- 8 green onions, chopped

- 8 teaspoons of Worcestershire sauce

- 4 tablespoons of balsamic vinegar

- 4 tablespoons of soy sauce

How to Make It:

In a medium bowl, mix the Worcestershire sauce, soy sauce and balsamic vinegar together until combined. Place the beef in the bowl and allow to marinate for 2 hours. It will taste better and be more tender the longer you marinate it. If possible, you can place the beef in the marinade the night before.

When ready to prepare the meal, heat a wok until it is hot. Do not add any oil to the wok. Add beef and the marinade to the skillet and allow to cook until beef is completely cooked. Add the vegetables to the beef in the wok and allow to stir fry for an addition 2-3 minutes. You can add a bit of water if the stir fry begins sticking to the pan. If you have too many ingredients to fit well in your wok, you can do this in batches.

Place the stir fried meat and veggies in a large serving bowl. Divide into four servings and serve while warm. Enjoy. Makes 4 servings.

Grilled Apricot Pork Skewers Recipe

You do not have to resort to bland, boring foods when you are doing your fasting days for your intermittent fasting diet. Instead, you should focus on delicious healthy foods that are packed with yummy flavors. While it can seem tough to stick to your calorie restrictions, these skewers only pack about 285 calories per serving, so you can fit this delicious main dish into your fasting day without a problem. It is a simple recipe, making it perfect for a busy evening.

What You'll Need:

- 1 1/3 cups of chunked pork tenderloin, lean

- 16 pieces of dried apricots

- 1 tablespoon of olive oil

- Salt and pepper to taste

How to Make It:

Bring a couple cups of water to a boil. Place the dried apricots in a medium bowl. Pour the boiling water over the apricots until they are just covered with the boiling water. Allow them to soak in the boiling water for about 15 minutes to soften them.

Sprinkle pork chunks with some salt and rub into the

meat carefully.

Preheat your grill on medium heat, placing a grill pan on the grill to preheat as well.

Using 8 skewers, place apricots and pork chunks alternately on skewers, leaving a bit of room between the apricots and pork so they will cook well on the grill. Use a brush to brush skewers with a bit of olive oil. Place your skewers on the grill pan and allow to grill. They should grill for about eight minutes per side, but check to make sure that pork completely cooks through. Allow skewers to rest before you serve them. Eat while warm. Makes 4 servings.

NOTE: If using wooden skewers, be sure to soak well before using them on the grill.

Teriyaki Grilled Veggie Tofu Kebabs Recipe

Tofu offers a great way to get lean protein and it is low in calories as well. The teriyaki sauce gives this tofu dish a nice oriental flavor if you love that kind of food. You should serve the kebabs over some cauliflower rice, which is extremely low in calories as well. It will not take you long to make this meal, but you should allow your tofu to marinate for a minimum of 20 minutes for the best results. This dish only has about 190 calories for each serving.

What You'll Need:

- 1 ¼ cups of tofu, firm, cubed

- ¾ cup of courgette, chunked

- 2 tablespoons of teriyaki sauce

- ¾ cup of baby sweetcorn, chunked

- 8 green onions, chopped

- ½ cup of red bell peppers, chunked

- Cauliflower rice

How to Make It:

In a shallow dish, mix up all the chopped veggies with the tofu. Add the teriyaki sauce and toss well. Cover and place in the refrigerator allowing it to marinate for a minimum of 20 minutes. Prepare your skewers if you are using wooden skewers by soaking for 20-30 minutes.

Preheat a grill with a grill pan on it to medium heat.

While the grill is preheating, thread the veggies and tofu on skewers, alternating the ingredients. Place the skewers on the grill, allowing to cook for about 9-11 minutes, turning from time to time for even cooking. Serve the kebabs hot over portions of cauliflower rice and enjoy. Makes 4 servings.

Cilantro Chili Chicken Quesadillas Recipe

Some people like to only consume a single meal while they are on a fasting day. If you like to have just one big meal, then this delicious recipe is for you. It has 500 calories per serving and is delicious. This recipe, inspired by a recipe from iFasters, allows you to have Mexican food, even while you are on a fasting day. The great part is that this tasty dish is so easy to make and comes together in no time. Not only does it only have 500 calories, but it packs in 34 grams of protein too.

What You'll Need:

- 8 8-inch flour tortillas

- 2 cups of shredded chicken breast

- 1 4-oz can of chopped green chilies, well drained

- ¼ cup of fresh cilantro, chopped

- 1 cup of shredded Mexican cheese, low-fat

How to Make It:

Preheat your grill to medium heat.

To make the quesadillas, mix together the chopped cilantro and the shredded chicken in a large bowl.

Take a piece of aluminum foil about 30x18 inches and

place 1 tortilla in the middle of it. Add ¼ of the chicken mixture, ¼ cup of cheese and a quarter of the chilies. Place a tortilla on top of it and then wrap the tortilla in the foil, making a packet for the tortilla. Make a couple piercings with a fork in the foil to allow steam to vent out. Continue with the rest of your quesadillas.

Place the foil packets on the preheated grill, placing them on a rack that is about six inches from the heat. Allow to grill for about 14-16 minutes, ensuring that the cheese in the quesadillas completely melts. Remove from the grill.

Cut quesadillas into triangles and serve up while warm. Enjoy immediately. Refrigerate any leftovers. Makes 4 servings.

NOTE: You could also place the quesadillas in the oven if you do not want to grill them.

Pita and Smoked Salmon Pizza Recipe

For about 195 calories, you can enjoy this delicious pita smoked salmon pizza. It is a fun twist on pizza that gives you plenty of lean protein, some fiber from the pita bread and a delicious dinner that will not use all your calories on your fasting days. This recipe makes a single serving, but you can double or triple it if you need to feed more than one person.

What You'll Need:

- ¼ cup of diced red onion

- 1 lemon wedge

- 1 tablespoon of low fat, chive and onion cream cheese

- 1 teaspoon of drained capers

- 1/8 cup of sliced smoked salmon

- Lettuce leaves

- Pinch of fresh dill

- 1 whole wheat pita

How to Make It:

Preheat your oven to 350F.

Place the pita on a baking tray and then spread the

cream cheese on the pita. Top with pieces of the smoked salmon, scattering them over the pita. Sprinkle the capers and red onion on the pizza. Place in the oven and allow to bake for about 10 minutes. The pita bread should become golden brown on the edges.

Serve the pizza while hot, garnishing with some freshly chopped ill a lemon wedge and a bit of lettuce on the side. Enjoy. Makes 1 serving.

Mushroom Garlic Chicken Recipe

Inspired by a recipe from Jemma Eat World, this recipe is wonderfully delicious and makes a perfect dinner when you are on a fasting day. Each serving of this recipe only has 250 calories, so you have room for snacks and a good breakfast when you serve this for dinner. The mushrooms are delicious and the cottage cheese makes a low fat gravy for your chicken while adding even more protein to the dish.

What You'll Need:

2 cups of cottage cheese, low fat

4 small chicken breasts

1 cup of mushrooms

8 cloves of garlic

How to Make It:

Start by peeling and mincing the garlic. Then, slice all of the mushrooms, making sure they are very thinly sliced. Heat a skillet on medium heat and add a bit of olive oil cooking spray to the pan. Place the mushrooms and garlic in the pan, sautéing until they become almost tender.

Meanwhile, slice the chicken into thin strips.

After mushrooms are fully cooked, remove from a pan and sit to the side. Add chicken to the hot skillet and allow it to cook until the chicken strips are fully cooked and golden brown. Make sure you cook on both sides.

After the chicken is fully cooked, add the mushrooms back to the skillet. Place the cottage cheese in the skillet as well and stir the ingredients together. Allow to cook for a few more minutes until you have a nice mushroom gravy. Serve immediately and enjoy while hot. Makes 4 servings.

Easy Portabella and Mozzarella Pizzas Recipe

This tasty pizza recipe uses mushroom caps instead of a traditional pizza crust, which allows you to enjoy the flavor of the pizza without all the calories that come with the crust. In fact, each mushroom pizza only has 88 calories, so it is a tasty meal that is very low in calories, although it definitely boasts plenty of delicious flavors. Make this recipe up for a delicious lunch, snack or even your dinner. The whole family will probably enjoy this tasty recipe.

What You'll Need:

- 4 large Portobello mushrooms for stuffing

- 1 cup of chopped peppers and onions

- 8 tablespoons of mozzarella cheese, fat free

- ¾ cup of tomato sauce

How to Make It:

Preheat the oven to 350F.

Carefully wash the mushroom caps, allowing them to thoroughly dry before you stuff them. Remove the insides so you can stuff them.

Spray a baking pan with olive oil cooking spray. Place the mushroom caps on the pan and spray them with a bit of the cooking spray as well. Place mushrooms in the oven, allowing to cook for five minutes at 350 before you stuff them.

Remove the mushrooms and place ¼ of the sauce in each cap. Divide the veggies and cheese among the caps as well. Place back in the oven, allowing to cook for about 15 minutes at 350 or until mushrooms are fully cooked and cheese is melted. Remove from the oven and serve while warm. Makes 4 servings.

Spinach and Smoked Salmon Roulade Recipe

For only 167 calories you can enjoy a serving of this delicious spinach and smoked salmon roulade. It tastes great and it looks amazing too because it is so colorful. While it gives you a wonderful low calorie meal to eat on fasting days, it is so delicious that it makes a great recipe to make when you are having company, especially since it can be made in advance. For easy meals on fasting days, make it at the beginning of the week so it is prepared when you need it.

What You'll Need:

Spinach Cake Ingredients

- ½ cup of fresh parsley chopped

- 1/3 cup of flour

- 2 egg yolks, large

- Hot pepper sauce (dash)

- 10 ounces of frozen spinach, thawed and pressed dry

- ¼ cup of sour cream, reduced fat

- 6 egg whites, large

- Ground pepper and salt to taste

Filling Ingredients

- ¼ cup of fresh chives, chopped

- 3 tablespoons of rinse and drained capers

- ¾ cup of cottage cheese, low fat

- 8 ounces of flaked smoked salmon

- 6 ounces of cream cheese, reduced fat

- 1 tablespoon of lemon juice

- Pepper to taste

How to Make It:

Begin by preheating the oven to 375F. Prepare a baking sheet by lining with parchment paper and then spraying the parchment paper with olive oil cooking spray.

In a food processor, add hot pepper sauce, flour, spinach, sour cream and parsley. Process until you have a smooth mixture. Add a bit of pepper and salt. Add the egg yolks to the processor, pulsing until just mixed. Place the spinach mixture in a bowl and set to the side.

In a mixing bowl, beat egg whites until you begin to see stiff peaks form, but don't allow dry peaks to form. Place 1/3 of the whites into the spinach mixture and mix lightly with a spatula. Fold the remaining whites into the spinach mixture, only folding until just blended. Spread the mixture carefully in the pan that was already prepared. Bake for about 8-10 minutes or until the top is springy. Remove from the oven and allow to cook on a rack while in the pan for about 5-6 minutes.

Place a clean towel on your work surface. Carefully invert your spinach cake so it is on your towel. Remove the parchment paper and place another towel over the spinach cake.

Make the filling by adding the cottage cheese and cream cheese to a food processor. Process until you have a smooth mixture. Place in a small bowl and set to the side.

Take the towel off the spinach cake, sprinkling just a bit of lemon juice on the top of the cake. Spread half of your cream cheese mixture over the cake, leaving a border around all edges. Place salmon on top of the cream cheese mixture. Top with the rest of the cream cheese mixture. Sprinkle the capers and chives on top and season with a bit of black pepper.

Carefully begin rolling up the cake like a jelly roll, letting the towel help you as you roll it up. Use plastic wrap to completely wrap the roulade tightly so it does not unroll. Place in the refrigerator and refrigerate for 4 hours or overnight. Cut into 24 slices before serving. Serve 3 slices per person. Makes 8 3-slice servings. Enjoy!

Chapter 6: Fasting Diet Soups, Salads and Sandwiches

These soups, salads and sandwiches make wonderful lunches when you are following the intermittent diet. They are light and delicious, keeping your calorie intake down while keeping you full and your energy high. Some of these recipes are so tasty and filling that they make wonderful dinners as well. If you want a tasty salad, try the Tasty Thai Chicken Lime Salad or the Feta Cheese and Beet Salad. For a wonderful burger, the Tasty Turkey Burgers keep your burger low cal while making sure you get plenty of protein. Soups are easy on the stomach, making them a perfect choice for your fasting days, so consider trying the yummy Spanish Flavored Veggie and Fish Stew, or for a hot day, enjoy the Cool Gazpacho Soup.

Cabbage and Chicken Soup Recipe

For a 1-cup portion of this soup, you only take in 55 calories, so it is a wonderful recipe you can make for fasting days. In fact, if it is your dinner, you could have two cups of soup for only 110 calories, which helps you stay within your calorie range on a fasting day. You will get plenty of vegetables in the soup and the chicken breast ensures you get protein with this soup as well.

What You'll Need:

- 1 small onion, diced

- 2 bell peppers (any color) diced

- 1 teaspoon of thyme, dried

- 2 carrots, shredded

- 1 head of green cabbage, finely shredded

- Pepper and salt to taste

- 1 teaspoon of cayenne pepper (add more to taste if desired)

- 2 chicken bouillon cubes

- 1 chicken breast, skinless, boneless, chopped or shredded

How to Make It:

Dice or shred your chicken, placing it in a big saucepan or soup pot. Cover the chicken with water. Bring chicken and water to a boil, boiling the chicken for 30-35 minutes. When chicken is fully cooked, place the vegetables in the pot, adding more water if necessary to ensure all ingredients are covered. Add the bouillon cubes as well, ensuring they are completely mixed into the water. Allow to boil for 10 more minutes. Place the spices in the soup and mix well, allowing to cook for 2-3 more minutes. Serve up and enjoy while hot.

Makes 6 1-cup servings or 3 2-cup servings.

Tasty Turkey Burgers Recipe

You do not have to give up burgers, even on fasting days. You can have a burger and stick to your fasting diet too. These turkey burgers only have 175 calories per serving, so it will not take up all your calories when you are doing a fasting day. If you are willing to eat a few more calories, top the burgers with some low calorie tomato salsa.

What You'll Need:

- 2 cups of ground turkey

- 4 cloves of garlic, minced

- 2 teaspoons of ground coriander

- 3-4 green onions, chopped finely

- 2 teaspoons of ground cumin

- 2 red chilies, seeds and stem removed, chopped finely

- 2 large eggs, beaten (add enough to make the mixture stick together)

How to Make It:

In a large bowl, combine the ground turkey, garlic, coriander, green onions, cumin and chilies. Mix well. Place in the refrigerator allowing the flavors to combine, allowing to marinate for at least 30 minutes. When done marinating, add the eggs to the mixture, only adding enough to make the mixture stick together. Make into four large patties.

Preheat the grill on medium heat. Place the patties on the preheated grill, allowing to grill for about 7-9 minutes per side, ensuring that they are cooked completely through. Remove from the grill. Serve up with some tomato salsa if desired. Makes 4 servings.

Feta Cheese and Beet Salad Recipe

When you want a low calorie, but tasty, salad, this salad is a great pick. Eat a whole serving for just 204 calories, which helps you keep calorie counts low for the day. It makes it easy to stick to your fasting diet when you can make such delicious, easy fasting diet recipes. The combination of steamed beets and feta is delicious and the lemon juice adds a nice zing to the salad.

What You'll Need:

- 10 ounces of spinach or mixed greens of choice

- 2 teaspoons of lemon juice

- 20 beet roots, medium sized

- ¾ cup of crumbled Feta cheese

- 2 teaspoons of olive oil

- Pepper to taste

- 2 small red onions, diced

How to Make It:

Carefully clean off the beets, but avoid over peeling or over scrubbing them. Cut the beets into ¼ inch pieces and then place in a pot of boiling water or a steamer. Steam the beets until they become tender. Strain the beats and allow them to fully dry and cool off.

Meanwhile, mix the pepper, lemon juice and olive oil in a small bowl, whisking together thoroughly.

On four plates, spread the salad ingredients on four plates. Sprinkle each salad with ¼ of the red onions. Top with the beets and then sprinkle with the Feta cheese. Drizzle each salad with some of the lemon juice dressing and serve immediately while the beets are still a bit warm. Makes 4 servings.

Turkey and Vegetable Soup Recipe

This recipe is inspired by a recipe from About.com's Low Fat cooking section and offers a delicious soup that is full of flavor while very low in calories. One serving of the soup only has 111 calories, so you will not blow your calories all in one shot with this recipe. It makes it easy to stick to your calorie restrictions when adding this soup to your fasting days.

What You'll Need:

- 1 stalk of celery, chopped

- ½ cup of brown rice, uncooked

- 1 cup of shredded turkey

- 6 cups of chicken broth, fat free

- 1 carrot, chopped

- Salt and pepper to taste

How to Make It:

In a large saucepan, place the broth and turn the heat on high, bringing it to a boil. Once it is boiling, reduce the heat until the broth is simmering gently. Place the rice, celery and carrots in the pan. Allow to simmer while covered for 20-25 minutes, or until the rice is fully cooked and the veggies are completely tender. Place the shredded turkey into the saucepan, allowing it to cook for about 5-7 more minutes or until turkey is heated through. Add salt and pepper to taste. Serve hot. Makes 6 servings.

Cool Gazpacho Soup Recipe

When the temperature begins to soar, a nice, cool dinner is the perfect way to end a long, hot day. Gazpacho is the perfect choice, since it is tasty and refreshing. Not only does it offer a cool, refreshing dish to serve on a hot day, but it is a low calorie soup that makes a great addition to your fasting days. It is very easy to make, so you will not have to spend a lot of time working in the kitchen to prepare a nice meal. One serving of this gazpacho is only 100 calories.

What You'll Need:

- 6 tablespoons of orange juice, freshly squeezed

- 4 cloves of garlic, minced

- 2 red bell peppers, seeds and stem removed, chopped roughly

- 2 yellow onions, chopped roughly

- 2 jalapenos, seeds and stems removed, chopped roughly

- 2 large cucumbers, peeled and chopped roughly (remove seeds too)

- 6 pounds of tomatoes, cores removed and chopped roughly

- Sea salt and pepper to taste

How to Make It:

In a large bowl, combine the garlic, red bell peppers, jalapenos, onions, cucumbers and tomatoes. In smaller batches, place part of the veggie mix in a food processor and process until smooth. If needed, add a small amount of water if the mixture becomes too thick. Continue until all the veggies have been processed. Use a sieve and strain processed veggies to make sure any solids are removed. Place pureed veggies in a large bowl, adding the salt, pepper and orange juice. Mix well.

Place the soup in the refrigerate. Allow to chill for at least a couple hours before you serve it. Serve cold and garnish with a bit of sliced cucumber if desired. Makes 8 servings.

Tasty Thai Chicken Lime Salad Recipe

Sometimes salads can get a bit boring, but this salad uses unique flavors to make sure you get a unique salad that will tempt your taste buds. At only 143 calories per serving, you can easily add this salad to your meals on a fasting day. If has a nice combination of flavors, including delicious red chilies and lime juice. Once you make this tasty salad, you will definitely want to make it again.

What You'll Need:

- 8 green onions, finely chopped

- ¾ cup of shredded or diced chicken, cooked

- 2 cloves of garlic, minced

- 3 ounces of iceberg lettuce leaves, left whole

- 2 red chilies, chopped finely and seeds removed

- Mint sprigs to taste

- Diced coriander leaves, 2 handfuls

- 2 squeezes of lime juice

How to Make It:

Divide the iceberg leaves among two salad plates.

In a small bowl, mix the coriander leaves, garlic, chilies, onion and mint leaves. Mix well. Add the lime juice and toss again. Place meat in the bowl and toss until the meat is coated with the mixture. Divide the mixture between the two plates, using it to top the leaves of iceberg lettuce. Eat immediately. Makes 2 servings.

Chapter 9: Fasting Diet 10 Day Meal Plan

If you are fairly new to the fasting diet, it can be tough at first to get into the habit of following those two fasting days during the week. According to the intermittent diet, the fasting days should not be consecutive, so you will not feel like you are depriving yourself while following the diet. To help you get the 5:2 plan down pat, we've created an easy fasting diet 10 day meal plan that you can follow to get you started. For the fasting days, we've plugged in some of our great recipes and ensured that you do not get more than your 500-600 calories on the fasting day. On the other days, you can eat whatever you enjoy eating. Try using this meal plan to make sure you get started out the right way, increasing your intermittent fasting diet results. You can use the plan and plug in other recipes in the book as well if you want some variation.

Day 1:

Eat normally!

Day 2:

Fasting Day

Breakfast: Egg White and Spinach Omelet Recipe (80 calories)

Lunch: Tasty Turkey Burgers Recipe (175 calories)

Dinner: Grilled Apricot Pork Skewers Recipe (285 calories)

TOTAL: 540 calories

Day 3:

Eat Normally!

Day 4:

Eat Normally!

Day 5:

Fasting Day

Breakfast: Berry Blend and Banana Breakfast Smoothie Recipe (126 calories)

Snack: Glazed and Iced Cinnamon Pineapple Dessert Recipe (160 calories)

Dinner: Beef and Veggie Stir Fry Recipe (260 calories)

TOTAL: 546 calories

Day 6:

Eat Normally!

Day 7:

Eat Normally!

Day 8:

Fasting Day

Breakfast: Tasty Bran Banana Muffins Recipe (97 calories)

Lunch: Cabbage and Chicken Soup Recipe (55 calories)

Dinner: Mushroom Garlic Chicken Recipe (250 calories)

Snack: Lemon and Blueberry Yogurt Cake Recipe (115 calories)

TOTAL: 517 calories

Day 9:

Eat Normally!

Day 10:

Fasting Day

Breakfast: Poached Eggs with Asparagus Breakfast Recipe (150 calories)

Lunch: Turkey and Vegetable Soup Recipe (111 calories)

Snack: Tasty Veggie and Cheese Stuffed Mushrooms Recipe (79 calories)

Dinner: Low Cal Turkey Bolognese Recipe (182 calories)

TOTAL: 522 calories

www.ingramcontent.com/pod-product-compliance
Ingram Content Group UK Ltd.
Pitfield, Milton Keynes, MK11 3LW, UK
UKHW020138250726
13967UKWH00002B/736

9 781633 830615